GOD'S HEALING

FOR YOUR TRAUMA

A Personal Journey

Jerry Brecheisen

God's Healing for the Traumas of Life: A Personal Journey
ISBN: 0-9716100-2-9

Copyright © 2001, 2006
by Loren G. Brecheisen
Library of Congress: 2006903613

Published by: Brecksong Publications
Brecksong, LLC
PO Box 6073
Fishers, IN 46038
317.578.2398
jerry@brecksong.com
www.brecksong.com

Printed in the United States of America. All rights reserved under International Copyright Law. Contents and/or cover may not be reproduced in whole or in part in any form without the express written consent of the Publisher.

Cover Design: Lyn Rayn
Photo: Jerry Brecheisen

All Scripture quotations not otherwise designated are from the *Holy Bible, New International Version* (NIV). Copyright © 1973, 1978, 1984 by International Bible Society. Used by permission of Zondervan Publishing House. All rights reserved.

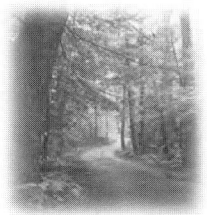

TABLE OF CONTENTS

Foreword	5
Preface	7
Remember, God Let It Happen	11
Consider Pain A Passageway	25
Determine To Win	35
Use Your Trauma To Teach Others	45
Focus On The Deliverance	55
Learn To Live Again	61
Turn Your Weakness Into Strength	73
Never Lose Your Sense of Worth	83
As Simple as A-B-C	91
Steps to Your New Life	93
How to Study the Bible	95

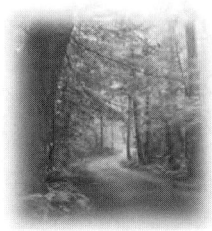

ACKNOWLEDGEMENTS

To Carol for her unfailing love and untiring support.

To Mandi and Arianna, my darling daughters.

To Ethel for always being there.

To Dad & Mom for unending prayers.

To Stan, my friend and brother.

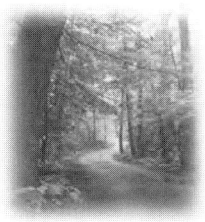

Foreword

Advice isn't advice, any more than "parts is parts." When you want to know how to do something, you look for someone with experience in the field. So, when you want some help for getting through a traumatic situation, you look for someone who is experienced. And it also helps if that person has personally overcome such a situation.

Obviously, you've picked up the right book. Jerry Brecheisen is truly an overcomer. He has been a friend of mine for over 25 years and I know, firsthand, of his overcoming a life-threatening illness and major surgery. However, he'll be the first to say that he didn't do it alone. Jerry learned to rely on the power and promises of God. And he experienced God's healing in such a way that it has given him personal victory not only over the illness and surgery itself, but also over its long-term effects.

God's Healing for Your Trauma: A Personal Journey is filled with practical advice for anyone going through a crisis, or for anyone in the recovery process. It's written with Jerry's characteristic humor, and yet it addresses the very serious issues of life in a thoughtful and compassionate way.

This revised edition of his book, *Turning Your Trauma Into Triumph*, is smaller in size but certainly not in content. It was a great source of help and healing when my wife, Linda, was going through a bout with colon cancer.

I pray that you will not only read it and apply its truths to your own life, but I also pray that you will pass it along. You probably know someone right now who needs to see how the weakness resulting from a traumatic situation can actually be turned into strength.

You may have heard Jerry give his testimony in person. If so, you know that the advice in this book comes straight from his heart. He has lived his message, and that makes a world of difference.

- Stan Toler

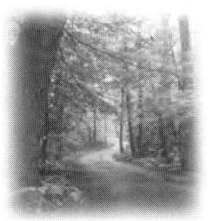

PREFACE

A doctor told the true story of a 78-year-old patient. After examining the man, the doctor recommended that he come back in six months for another check-up. The patient slowly shook his head and said to his physician, "Doctor, I won't be here in six months."

The doctor was stunned, but he put his arm around the man's shoulders and with a kindly smile he said, "Friend, you'll be around for a long time."

"No sir," the man replied, "I won't be here in six months. I'll be in Florida. I go there every year at that time!"

Working Principles For Unpredictable Problems

Some things aren't quite as predictable. A sudden hospitalization and a major surgery made a shambles of my schedule, and quicker than a Tsetse fly in a tornado, my whole world turned upside down. But God turned it right side up. And in the process I discovered eight workable principles for realizing God's healing in the traumas of life.

- How do I know they work?

- They worked when the doctor said I might not make it through the surgery.

- They worked when I had full cardiac arrest during a routine hospital procedure, and had an out-of-body experience.

- They worked when I had to learn how to walk again.

- They worked when facial paralysis drastically altered my appearance.

- They worked when I had to cope with mental depression and frustrating physical limitations.

I discovered that a mighty God isn't intimidated by our traumas. His sovereign purpose can grow stately trees of mercy from the painfully-cultivated soil of our lives.

Oswald Chambers said: "Faith must be tested because it can be turned into personal possession only through conflict." And it became a personal possession. Even as I hovered over the hospital bed where medical attendants were trying to re-start my heart, I settled into the strong arms of a Heavenly Father. In the darkest hours of my life, I made the discovery that God's light at its dimmest is infinitely brighter than trauma's shadow at its darkest.

Great Inevitability, Great Deliverance

If you haven't already gone through some sort of trauma, you probably will. It's the great inevitability. Ever since

Adam and Eve's rebellion in the Garden of Eden, trouble has dogged the human race like horseflies at a Sunday school picnic.

If your trouble isn't in a hospital room, then it might be in a funeral chapel, courtroom, anger-filled living room, or anywhere else where life is at its worst.

This book isn't some cutesy cure-all. Only God is in control of the cures!

This is a personal journal—a testimony of God's deliverance that I pray will encourage your heart *in the midst of it all*. Whether you're hanging from the rafters of rapture over some great and yet bewildering victory or agonizing over the ash heap of some awful adversity, this book is intended to give you a hook on which you can hang a spiritual hat.

It's said that Renoir, the famed artist, suffered excruciatingly from arthritis. His hands often gnarled and cramped as he suffered to even hold a paintbrush. As his friend watched the ordeal and yet marveled at the developing masterpiece on the canvas, he remarked, "Why do you persist, with such pain?"

The painter replied, "Ah, my friend, the pain passes but the beauty remains."

Amen!

Same Truth, New Package

This is a revised edition of a previous book. I have added a few thoughts but I've tried to keep most of the message that so many of you have commented about. Your letters and personal words of encouragement about that book have warmed my soul.

I don't know what you're going through, but I know who will take you through!

Several years have gone by since the first writing. But the promises and power of God are eternal. Unshaken by disease, destruction, or division, His perfect Word and His perfect will continue to wind their way through the deserts of life, with supernatural refreshment.

God's healing is *still* the solution for your trauma.

– Jerry Brecheisen

ONE

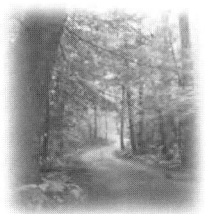

REMEMBER, GOD LET IT HAPPEN

What then shall we say?
Is God unjust? Not at all!
(Romans 9:14)

The nurse told me he was coming to give me one of those "doctor talks" before my surgery in the morning. But when I saw Dr. Volkel walk through the door, I had an uneasy feeling. As he began the conversation, I began to separate polite courtesy from the concern scrawled on his face in thin lines.

With surgical skill, he cut through the casual and went straight for the facts.

"Jerry, you have a benign tumor on the auditory nerve near the brain. It's called an Acoustic Neuroma. We don't understand where they come from and how they grow, but we need to remove it immediately. If we don't, you could suffer a cerebral hemorrhage."

Suddenly it got as quiet as an Amish rock concert.

The word "benign" wrapped itself around my mind like a warm blanket, but "brain," "tumor," and "immediately" brought a chill to my bones. I just couldn't believe this was happening. The symptoms had been perplexing—slight hearing loss, dizziness, vertigo, one king-size headache—but to think I was facing a major surgery in just a few hours was mind-boggling.

He continued methodically but compassionately, "It will be a very lengthy surgery. You'll be asleep and placed in an upright position. We'll shave your head and then open your skull with a semi-circular incision to allow us access to the tumor."

The more he talked, the more I realized this was serious stuff! A thousand questions orbited my mind.

"Open your skull . . ." *What if you can't get it back together?*
"Shave your head . . ." *Will my hair grow back?*
"Get to the tumor . . ." *What kind of a vegetable would I be?*

Fear was probably written on my face like a neon "OPEN" sign in an all-night diner. He patted my arm and began to answer questions I didn't even have enough presence of mind to ask. Soon, the "doctor expression" crept into his eyes and he said, "It's a very serious surgery and there is a chance you will not survive." He talked about "fifty/fifty," but I would later learn he was thinking more about "eighty/twenty" (against!).

Don't Be Afraid of the Big "W"

I listened to the details with more attention than a sweat bee at a Weight Watchers convention. "Once we get you through the surgery you'll be going to intensive care for several days. After that, you'll be moved to your own room and go through several weeks of therapy."

The word "therapy" brought a slight ray of sunshine into a room that was growing increasingly cloudy. I actually looked forward to it when I began to consider the alternatives.

"You won't be aware of anything for many hours, or even several days." Dr. Volkel continued, "Do you have any questions?"

Yes, I thought to myself. *One question: WHY?* I had heard "The Big W" many times as a pastor, when I stood with loved ones in funeral chapels and hospital rooms. Now it was making the rounds of my own spirit. As he started to leave I asked, "Doctor, what are the implications of this surgery?"

Slowly, he came back and sat in the steel chair next to my bed and began to explain:

I would suffer a total loss of hearing in my left ear. *What about singing and hearing the pitch of a song?*

The tear duct in my left eye would be affected, leaving me with a dry eye. *How would that alter my appearance?*

My motor skills would be affected. *Will I be able to play the piano again?*

Then he threw in the kicker. "A facial nerve is involved, and there will likely be a drooping of the left side of your mouth." I imagined how that would look as I stood behind the pulpit on Sunday morning! It wasn't a very good pep talk, but as I grew to know this esteemed neurosurgeon, I began to understand his professional need to paint the clouds with broader strokes then the sunbeams. His matter-of-fact attitude actually comforted me.

Little did I know then what the next several hours would hold! The surgery would stretch for nearly ten hours; my heart would stop during a routine change of bandages; I would have an "out-of-body" experience; almost every motor skill on the left side of my body would have to be re-learned. The big "W" would parade itself before my mind several times.

Did you ever whisper the word "Why?" under your breath? Or, have you ever screamed it at the top of your lungs?

Asking "Why?" doesn't mean that you're some spiritual reprobate. It merely certifies that you are a card-carrying member of the human race!

But here's the good news: God's grace and mercy aren't compromised by our questions.

And best of all, we're not the first to ask.

It fell from the lips of His own Son on the blood-spattered slope of Golgatha's hill.

> *About the ninth hour Jesus cried out in a loud voice, 'Eloi, Eloi, lama sabachthani?'—which means, 'My God, my God, why have you forsaken me?'* (Matthew 27:46)

The Great High Priest who was tempted in every way we are and yet without sin is touched by the feeling of our infirmity. *For we do not have a high priest who is unable to sympathize with our weaknesses, but we have one who has been tempted in every way, just as we are—yet was without sin* (Hebrews 4:15).

I love the story of the little grandson who was attending his first church service. Looking around the big sanctuary, he noticed the wooden cross on the wall behind the platform. He nudged his grandmother, and she bent to hear him. With cupped hands he whispered, "Grandma, why do they have these *plus signs* hanging all over the building?"

In fact, there are plus signs everywhere—even over the battlefields of your life. God, in His wise and wonderful providence, turned the awful agony of the Cross into a glorious advantage.

He let *that* happen to bring salvation and healing to your sin or sickness!

George Bennard's grand old gospel song says it so well:

> *In the old rugged cross, stained with blood so divine, a wondrous beauty I see; for 'twas on that old cross Jesus suffered and died to pardon and sanctify me.*
>
> *So I'll cherish the old rugged cross, till my trophies at last I lay down. I will cling to the old rugged cross, and exchange it someday for a crown.*

It's said that Dr. Billy Graham entered a packed room at a University of Minnesota student-faculty meeting and remarked that many had come just out of curiosity. Smiling, he added, "I can always count on the department of psychology showing up in full force."

So can we. Trauma affects every area of our lives—including the psychological. God created us with an emotional capacity that includes fears and questions. And the Enemy of our faith, whose sole purpose is to "kill, steal, and destroy," loves to erect flimsy tents of spiritual doubt over our rock-solid, and very human, questions.

Take Another Look At That Question Mark

It's also worth noting that the question mark of Calvary ("Why?") turned to a great exclamation point. *When he had received the drink, Jesus said, 'It is finished.' With that, he bowed his head and gave up his spirit* (John 19:30). Heaven was in control to the very last. Nobody "took" Jesus' spirit. He "gave up" His spirit. The question was merely a prelude to the conquest!

"It is finished!" The cause of salvation is won!
Buds of mercy and healing grew from the splattered soil!
Healing is forever provided!
Heaven won and hell lost!

Take another look at that question mark in your life. Notice that it has a bow in it (?). I've discovered that the bow in the question mark (?) is simply an exclamation point (!) with a God-planned detour.

Even in the question marks of your life the exclamation points of God's power and presence are always there beneath the surface!

He knows the way—He's been there before.

He will not fail you when the times cover your soul like a wet woolen blanket.

There's a plus sign in the room! I discovered that firsthand.

Life is a Training Ground for Trauma

Dr. Volkel left my hospital room as politely as he had arrived, but I was not the same. My thoughts traversed the miles from the hospital to a church parsonage. There, my dear wife, Carol, who was expecting our first child, would anticipate the doctor's talk and the subsequent surgery. The tests, the sudden hospitalization, and the impending surgery had been difficult for her. Graced with kindness and compassion, Carol had always been able to cope with her own pain, but hated to see others suffer.

I knew she would want to hear all the details. *Now . . . if I could just remember them!* I'll have to confess that my thinking that night was not quite as sharp as I hoped the scalpel would be in the morning! (And I was also trying to figure out a way to take up an offering in the hospital to meet the surgeon's fee.)

I thought about our church. We were so young and inexperienced, and yet we were responsible for one of the oldest congregations in our denomination. Our first church was "blessed" with a "senior" pastor who was only twenty-two years old. I'm sure they restrained themselves from patting me on the head and saying, "Nice little talk, Junior," as they departed from the morning worship each week.

Some of them went out of their way to make our first pastoral experience a "growing experience," while others wrapped their arms of love, understanding, and acceptance around us. We would learn to feel the strength of that embrace throughout the next year.

I thought of my family. I could only imagine the heaviness of their hearts as they got the call to come to my bedside.

For years, the Brecheisen family had shared the awesome along with the awful, traveling coast-to-coast in a gospel music ministry. We had the opportunity to see the USA, as few others would ever see it. Love and faith was the glue that held us together. This would be no exception!

Life "on the road" was a great training ground for the traumas of life that would come later. As a matter of fact, as we look at our traumas we'll discover that we've been in training for them throughout our lives.

As it all played on the monitor of my mind, I knew that it was a night for which sleeping pills were born.

God Always Answers in Person

After my family left, I gathered my wilted wits and the facsimile of a dressing gown around me, and took the longest walk of my life. The hospital corridor was jammed with silver carts, wooden chairs, and plastic receptacles—monuments of mercy in a desert of despair.

White-robed messengers scurried about, filling out their aluminum-covered flip charts, as they answered numerous call-buttons. And blue uniformed maintenance crews tried valiantly to smooth the wake they left behind. Through the ceiling speakers, switchboard operators chided various doctors for not answering their calls.

But no one seemed to notice the weary wanderings of one patient who faced a morning surgery.

I was alone.

As alone as I had ever felt in the previous twenty-two years of my life. The Apostle John's New Testament isle of Patmos was surely a teeming metropolis, compared to the echoing emptiness of that hallway.

What races through the mind of one who has given himself to stand beside the hurts of others as a minister of the gospel, as he faces his own crisis? I can only speak for myself.

I thought about my relationship with God. At that moment nothing but the eternal destiny of my own soul mattered. It was my turn to face the platform of the heavens and ask silent questions that only the Holy Spirit could answer:

Why me? Why this? Why now?

They were questions I suddenly wasn't afraid to ask. A sign in a Chicago store read, "I have been in this business a long time. I have been cussed and discussed; talked about and lied to; I have been taken for granted and taken to the cleaners; I have been looked over and stepped on. Matter of fact, the only reason I am staying in business now is to see WHAT IN THE WORLD IS GOING TO HAPPEN TO ME NEXT!"

Some of the great struggles of time haven't been waged on the fields of Gettysburg or the rocks of Normandy. They have taken place in hospital rooms, divorce courts, and prison cells.

There, finite, created humans have mind-wrestled with the sovereign purposes of the Creator and wondered, "What next?"

The New Testament leader, Paul, addressed such people in his letter to Roman Christians. After suffering under pagan authorities, they were just waiting to see what would happen next. Some of them thought they deserved only sunny days and starry nights. In the midst of it all, the apostle takes them to the school of God's sovereignty.

"Sovereign" is said to come from the root word "Super"—free from outside control, supreme jurisdiction or dominion. Paul wrote,

> *But who are you, O man, to talk back to God? 'Shall what is formed say to him who formed it, 'Why did you make me like this?' Does not the potter have the right to make out of the same lump of clay some pottery for noble purposes and some for common use?* (Romans 9:20-21).

God's will is the hinge to the door of faith. Because He is sovereign, He has the right to cause or allow anything in the lives of those whom He created, without compromising His character or His loving purpose. He inspects every detail and stamps it "Holy and Just." Anything else would be out of character.

Several years ago I took my family to see the breathtaking beauty of a northern Michigan falls. The journey to the falls was tiring and the "Are-we-there-yets" of our darling daughters, Mandi and Arianna, added to the challenge. What seemed to be hours (but was probably only minutes) along a stony path to the falls was worth every effort *when we finally arrived.*

There, like a scene from the Travel Channel, a summer sun kissed the blue forehead of that river until it swooned in white-foamed ecstasy over the falls. And all of its gracefulness happened in front of the massive, beautiful tangle of an evergreen forest. We could only stand in awe.

Similarly, graceful streams of mercy run past the tangled forests of our lives. James, the Lord's earthly brother, added, *The wisdom that comes from heaven is first of all pure; then peace-loving, considerate, submissive, full of mercy and good fruit, impartial and sincere* (James 3:17).

God's way is *perfectly* perfect.

He let it happen. And everything He appoints or allows is a reflection of that perfection. Somewhere, in the outer regions of eternity, a heavenly huddle between the Father, Son, and Holy Spirit concluded that my surgery and all of its accompanying effects was the absolute best way.

But He didn't just leave me with the predicament. He came to me with His presence. In the awful silence of that hospital corridor, His Spirit sang a familiar hymn to my spirit:

> *The soul that on Jesus hath leaned for repose, I will not, I will not desert to his foes; that soul, tho' all hell should endeavor to shake, I'll never, no never, no never forsake.*

I was going to take a painful journey past tangled forests just like those behind the falls. But in person, God reminded me that the wonderful streams of His supply would always be available.

Your journey is often stony.

You tire.

But your *arrival* will reveal a splendor that will cause the soul to shout ten thousand "Hallelujahs!"

Here's where it begins: God let this happen! Your agreement with God's final control is the beginning of healing. Your acknowledgment that He can make a miracle out of a mess becomes the river of mercy that runs past the tangled forests.

God's absolute authority demands your absolute agreement.

That's where the peace comes from. When you resign yourself to say, "A loving God let this happen," you will have discovered the splendor at the end of the stony path.

John Wesley was once asked what he would do if he knew he would die at midnight. He replied, "I would retire to my room at 10 o'clock, commend myself to my heavenly Father, lie down to rest, and wake up in glory."

God spoke that kind of peace to my soul on my way back to my room.

And in those moments I knew that I was:

- Faulty but forgiven,
- Anxious but accepted,
- Lonely but not lost.

The 19th century lyrics of Lidie Edmunds is a firm reminder,

> *My faith has found a resting place, not in device nor creed; I trust the Everliving One, His wounds for me shall plead. Enough for me that Jesus saves, this ends my fear and doubt; A sinful soul, I came to Him, He'll never cast me out. My Great Physician heals the sick, the lost He came to save; For me His precious blood He shed, for me His life He gave.*

Let God Make a Miracle Out of a Mess

I can't comprehend how being stuck with needles and stitched with staples can be used in healing. But they can. God can make an advantage out of an adversity.

He can make . . .

> Character out of a car wreck
>
> Life out of a layoff
>
> Firmness out of an illness
>
> Tenacity out of a tear
>
> Peace out of a problem

Why? Because He is an all-knowing, all-powerful God who can be trusted with the details of our lives.

George Matheson wrote: "Make me a captive, Lord, and then I shall be free/Force me to render up my sword, and I shall conqueror be/I sink in life's alarm when by myself I stand/Imprison me within Thine arms, and strong shall be my stand."

It's a hope so great that if Madison Avenue could market it, its worth would leap from the tallest Dow Jones.

If the Metropolitan Opera could perform it, no amphitheater on earth could hold the crowd.

If Nashville could hum it, there wouldn't be enough studios to record it.

If the NFL could run with it, the fastest of earth could never tackle it.

But Jesus bought it for each of us on the awful ugliness of a wooden beam, raised above the sinful intents of false accusers. *For it is by grace you have been saved, through faith—and this not from yourselves, it is the gift of God—not by works, so that no one can boast* (Ephesians 2:8, 9).

It was a hope born on Calvary's hill overlooking a garbage dump near Jerusalem.

Alone with my Lord, I realized that every earthly effort meant little, compared to the moment I knelt and invited the Creator of Eternity to dwell in my earthly heart.

One of my favorite stories is of a Christian who quoted her favorite scripture verse as she lay dying: "I know whom I have believed, and am persuaded that He is able to keep that which I have committed unto Him against that day." Soon her strength failed and she was left with only a whisper that was clearly heard by everyone in the room, "I know."

And I knew! Had it not been for my pride and dignity (or whatever was left of it in that hospital gown), I would have brought the busyness of that hospital to a screeching halt with a shout, "I KNOW!"

God was in all of this. He'd make a miracle out of a mess.

His power would not be exhausted by a multi-hour surgery. A shaved head and a crooked mouth wouldn't alter His acceptance of me. His grace would not be tempered by the taunts of hell's messengers. His love would not be distanced by the closed doors of an elevator on the journey to an operating room.

God let it happen.

Learn that deep in your spirit. God sees some heavenly way to bring His sovereign purpose of love, peace, and holiness into the tangled forests of your life so that at the end of the journey, you might glimpse the beauty and splendor of it all.

Fellow airline passengers asked a little boy if he was afraid of the thunderstorm that was buffeting the plane. "Oh, no sir," he replied, "You see, my dad's the pilot and he's been through a lot bigger storms than this!"

The psalmist David didn't take too many airplane rides but he had confidence in a Heavenly Father who had no fear of the storms in his life.

> *You are a shield around me, O LORD; you bestow glory on me and lift up my head. To the LORD I cry aloud, and he answers me from his holy hill. I lie down and sleep; I wake again, because the LORD sustains me. I will not fear the tens of thousands drawn up against me on every side* (Psalm 3:3-6).

Was God unrighteous to allow this surgery to come into the lives of a young pastor and his family? Certainly not.

I can't say that church bells were ringing in my heart. I faced the longest day of my life and I knew it. I faced an altered way of living. I faced the uncertainty of a night without an earthly dawn.

But the trip back to my room was lighter. I had wrestled with my doubts and the Holy Spirit had won. He had spoken the peace of Jesus to my soul.

I lay me down to sleep and KNEW the Lord my soul would keep.

Then came the morning.

TWO

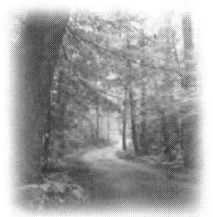

CONSIDER PAIN A PASSAGEWAY

'LORD,' Martha said to Jesus, 'if you had been here, my brother would not have died. But I know that even now God will give you whatever you ask'
(John 11:21-22).

The lights came on early surgery morning. My lovely wife held my hand and gave me one of those wonderful, "Everything will be all right" looks. Other family members were there, supporting me with their prayers and presence, but no one could take the place of that redheaded homecoming queen from Elkton, Michigan, whose glorious giggle lit up every room she ever entered.

We had shared so much in our young ministry. But this was *D-Day,* and the forces of the enemy would try to forever still the voice of a young preacher and steal the smile from his faithful wife. I silently prayed that God would give her strength for the ordeal.

It was an "Even now" event.

Soon I was wearing one of those lovely back-less hospital gowns and that cute little hair net, waiting for my limo to take me to surgery. Little did I know it would be a gurney that had been stored in the freezer!

Life Is In The Now

Martha said to the Master, "Even now . . . "

Life is full of "Even now" events.

"Before" is a word that brings wonderful memories of more contented days—roaring fires, soft snows, meadows ablaze with golden wildflowers, jumping into a beckoning pile of autumn leaves.

"Later" is a word that springs eternal—dreams of a retirement home, a promised promotion, cruise ships sailing out of penny jar savings, visions of a walk down the aisle, or a proud stride across a graduation platform.

But life is in the "now." It includes the tears as well as the tulips.

It includes the bitter along with the beautiful.

It runs the gauntlet from happiness to heartache, fruition to frustration.

Martha, Mary, and Lazarus were close friends of Jesus, in Bible times. Lazarus had died. His sister was brokenhearted when she reported it to the Master. "If you had been here, things would have been different," she reminded.

Her next words were full of faith. "But I know that *even now* God will give you whatever you ask." The Son of God had laid aside the power that He enjoyed before coming to earth, and depended on the authority and provision of His Heavenly Father during His redemptive sojourn.

"Even now . . . "

"Even now, you can make a difference, Jesus." For Martha, this painful moment was merely a passageway for His glory. The Lord Jesus Christ wasn't helpless at her hurts. Only moments later His voice would crush the stillness of the graveyard with the words, "Lazarus, come forth!"

It's easier to trust the Lord with our "Befores" and "Laters" than it is with our "Nows." But He is the Lord of the NOW—the "same yesterday, today, and forever."

Turning My "Hills Unto The Eyes"

"It's time," the nurse said, as the gurney was rolled into the room by those orderlies wearing mosquito-net hats.

There was still a wonderful peace within our hearts.

We would not question God's timing. "Even now" He would care for His own. "Even now" He could turn our crisis into His cause. "Even now" we would trust Him.

Hugs, kisses, and prayers were offered as I was placed on the gurney.

Dad walked by me as far as he could. I thought he showed more courage than I could have shown if my firstborn were being wheeled away for such serious surgery. He patted me on the arm and quoted a verse of scripture. "Remember Son, the Bible says, 'I will lift up my hills unto the eyes.'" It wasn't exactly a direct quote from Psalm 121 but it was close enough, considering that tense situation.

Since then I've thought about that "misquote." First, it was a great icebreaker. Second, it was full of truth. The Brecheisen family was, in fact, lifting the "hills" of their lives unto God's eternally vigilant "eyes." Somebody said, "That'll preach."

The elevator ride was claustrophobic. Maybe that's the day

I decided that elevators and I would never be on friendly terms. I've been known to leave women and children stranded on elevators when the door opened just wide enough for a pastor to pass through. Almost without exception, whenever I get on a populated elevator someone will say something like, "Don't you just feel like the walls are closing in on you" or "I hope they've finally fixed this thing. It stopped twice last week." It almost never fails!

Upon my arrival in the operating room I was greeted by a less than friendly nurse. She was probably upset because she had to get up so early, and my attitude wasn't so great either, since I had missed my morning cup of coffee. At the prices most hospitals charge, I don't think coffee and doughnuts in the operating room is totally unreasonable!

The injected sedative quickly took affect and I was not only in God's hands, I was in the hands of medical talent whose abilities God had formed in His mind ten trillion years before the stars were born.

The writer to the Hebrews summed up heaven's presence in our predicaments: *'Never will I leave you; never will I forsake you'* (Hebrews 13:5).

"Even now" my Heavenly Father had the situation under control.

Prayer requests had been sent across denominational and state lines. (Still today, someone will occasionally come up to me and say, "We prayed for you at our church.") I was surrounded—completely engulfed in the grace and mercy of the divine. His angels were watching *over* me, His family was standing *alongside* me, and the Scripture was saying, "*underneath* are the everlasting arms."

My "historians" tell me the surgery was long and very

tedious. The tumor that had been seen as the size of a fifty-cent piece on X-ray was discovered to be the size of a lemon, once the incision was made. Today's equipment may have discovered the actual size. In fact, the entire surgery would not be so invasive today. Laser surgery has made it possible to excise benign tumors without such drastic procedures as those practiced when I had the surgery.

Healed — One Way Or Another

I firmly believe that, according to God's loving purpose, some will be healed instantaneously from sickness and disease. But I also believe that He sometimes uses the skills of dedicated medical personnel to bring about healing in the lives of His children. He used the latter in my life.

Dr. Voelkel performed over nine hours of surgery on me, working so close to the brain that a mere brush against a nerve caused my 48-hour bout of hiccups later in intensive care. And within an hour of the end of my surgery, he would be called on to perform brain surgery on the wife of his colleague, who had been severely injured in an auto accident. Thank God for dedicated doctors, nurses, and technicians!

Following surgery, Dr. Voelkel wearily but gently gathered my family together. It had been such a long day for them. They told me how patient and kind he was in sharing answers to their many questions.

They also told me of something he said that I wish I could have heard personally. As he faced my family and their obvious faith he confessed, "I am not a man of faith, but I felt as if someone was guiding my hand as I worked on Jerry."

Someone was!

And those who had so faithfully stood by thanked the

doctor. Then they gathered for prayer, to thank the Great Physician for my survival and to trust Him for the hours ahead.

"Even now" God had heard the prayer of faith.

Bad Stuff, Good People

Bad stuff does happen to good people. Job had his boils; David had his valley of the shadow of death; Jeremiah had his mud-filled cisterns; and Paul had his thorn in the flesh. But Jesus isn't crippled by our diseases or by our distresses!

His own wounds were for our victory. He will stand by us even when we can't stand. He is the Lord of the "Even nows."

During the surgery, my mother stood with her face toward a hospital window and pulled out a timeworn pocket Bible. She opened it "randomly" to Psalm 91 and the Holy Spirit spoke this promise to her heart from God's Word, *'Because he loves me,' says the Lord, 'I will rescue him; I will protect him, for he acknowledges my name. He will call upon me, and I will answer him; I will be with him in trouble, I will deliver him and honor him. With long life will I satisfy him and show him my salvation'* (Psalm 91:14-16).

Mother immediately drove a stake of faith into the ground of that promise. It was enough for her then and its enough for me, "Even *now*."

Code Blue

Following the surgery, I was moved to the forests of hanging IV tubes and green-lit monitors. One day later, during a routine change of bandages, I had a sudden seizure and went into full cardiac arrest. The "code blue" alarm was sounded and medical personnel raced toward intensive care, past my unsuspecting family. I can't imagine how they would've felt had they known those doctors and nurses were heading in my direction!

As usual, my "Senior Physician," Doctor Jesus, had it all worked out. A heart surgeon was checking on his patient in the bed next to mine when the bells and whistles announced my predicament. He had only to turn around to act as heaven's representative in my very human situation.

The View From Above

I don't know *how long* I was in cardiac arrest, but I do know *where I was*: up above the room, looking down on the situation! It was an "out-of-body" experience as real as the sunrise, and one that I didn't speak of until several years after the surgery.

I won't tell you that I went through heaven's portals, saw streets of gold, or Uncle Ralph's *Mansion Over the Hilltop*. I've read about such experiences and know, firsthand, that those reactions could be put together in the mind from the sights and sounds that surround the patient in a near-death situation.

My view from above was like looking through fog-covered glasses. I remember a slightly agitated feeling that my hands were bound. (Later I learned that my hands actually *were* bound to keep me from pulling the intravenous tube from my arm.) That momentary discomfort was the only disturbing feeling during the entire experience.

The most lasting sensation was one of seeing the brightest—and whitest—light I had ever seen. Interestingly, everyone who has a near-death experience sees the same light, as well as similar sights and sounds. The room was bathed in that light, except for a hazy opening through which I saw the medical personnel working on me.

Doctors and nurses surrounding my bed were trying to jump-start my heart, but I couldn't see their faces. The medical team seemed to be anxious but not frantic. The atmosphere was very calm and peaceful and I remember being at total peace, personally.

I heard a voice. It wasn't thunderous, but rather a calm, steady voice. It was a man's voice (sorry, ladies). He spoke in an authoritative, medium-range voice.

"Jerry, I have more for you to do."

I could write about being "touched by an angel," or some call to be a missionary. Or I could write about being given some supernatural plan to save the planet. But I won't, because it just didn't happen. In fact, almost everyone who has a near-death experience, hears *the same thing*.

What is that "step" people take during near-death? Is it "death's door" or some "green room" leading to the presence of the Righteous Judge? I don't know. In the New Testament story, from the "other side," the rich man told Lazarus (not Mary & Martha's brother) that there was a gulf between them. And Paul the apostle had a vision of a "third heaven" that leaves some questions about what's between the *first* and the *third*.

Naturally, there are some questions that will only be answered on my final trip!

I know I saw the light. I know I heard the voice. I know that I looked down from *some-where* and saw a definite *some-thing*. It's as real in my mind today as it was then.

Just Passing Through

The experience didn't last long. I remember a second level of calmness after hearing the voice—as if it were a familiar voice. I remember the ending. The light, the hazy opening, the forms around the bed, and the patient seemed to merge. Like "morphing" in a TV commercial, objects merged into other objects. Suddenly everything was in its proper perspective and my spirit seemed to be re-connected to my body.

The entire experience was a passageway. God led me through the psalmist's "valley of the shadow," to let me enjoy the tranquillity of "green pastures" and "still waters."

If Lazarus hadn't died, he wouldn't have experienced a resurrection.

If Lazarus hadn't died, Mary and Martha wouldn't have experienced heaven's comfort.

If Lazarus hadn't died, we wouldn't have seen the infinite power of God in the life of His Son.

Your own pain is such a passageway. You're going through (or you've been through) that situation ON PURPOSE. God is going to use this as a way to reveal His help, His holiness, and His loving plan for your life. That oft-quoted word of the prophet Jeremiah is just one indicator,

> *'For I know the plans I have for you,'* declares the LORD, *'plans to prosper you and not to harm you, plans to give you hope and a future'* (Jeremiah 29:11).

"Hope?" "Future?" These were words to Israel's *exiles* that were taken captive to Babylon. They must have been harder to swallow than a plate full of live shrimp! But they were true. God would do just as He said. The difficulty was in the trusting.

And speaking of faith . . . Faith in God's healing is always built on the foundation of the unseen. Hebrews 11:1 tells us: *Now faith is being sure of what we hope for and certain of what we do not see.*

"I just don't see any way . . . ."

Of course not! You can't see that far. God's passageways aren't built on the kilometers, miles, or yards of time. They stretch back and forth into eternity. For example, He built a sun so large and yet so far away that we can never reach it—or even look at it. Yet, its rays traverse space to warm the tiny petals of a daisy in that flower pot on the patio.

What an awesome passageway!

You're just "passing through." You're here (or you were there) on a temporary visa.

Your citizenship isn't in this strange land.

You may feel like that frazzled mother who was going through customs inspection after returning from a trip overseas. She had five kids, all under 10 years of age.

One was walking across the arms of the chairs in the waiting area.

Another was wrapping himself in the braided ropes of the walkway that he had disassembled.

The others were either crying or fighting.

The customs inspector said to the lady, "Madame, do you have any illegal drugs or weapons that you wish to declare?"

"Sir," the mother said angrily as she waved her hand toward her rebellious brood, "if I had any of those things, don't you think I would have used them by now!"

Drugs or weapons aren't equal to the fight. But God is. He can walk you through the dangers of this unfamiliar road and deliver you to a land where the sun always shines.

I had to trust Him during my days of recovery.

THREE

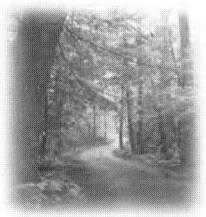

DETERMINE TO WIN

*He is like a tree planted by streams
of water, which yields its fruit in season
and whose leaf does not wither.
Whatever he does prospers*
(Psalm 1:3).

This artist had a bad back and suffered excruciating pain if he laid on it very long. He also had a nasal obstruction that hindered his air supply when lying in that position. But he laid on his back all day, every day, for 20 months. I've personally seen the results of that effort on the ceiling of the Cistine Chapel. Michelangelo was determined to get the job done.

The doctor expected me to stay in intensive care three weeks or more, but after 10 days, it was MOVING DAY! Now I was the new kid on the block of a four-bed ward.

I'm asked many times if I was in a lot of pain during the ordeal. The answer is no. Part of my miracle stay in intensive care was that it was pain free. Sedated to keep me from seizures, I was unaware that some of the hospital's most painful tests and procedures were conducted on me. Since I'm the type that might request a general anesthetic to get a haircut, it worked out just fine.

The Rigors of Recovery

The most painful procedures lay ahead.

They weren't in the form of needles; they were in the form of baby steps back to a full physical recovery. Everyone who has suffered a debilitating injury or sickness knows the frustration. Since motor skills were effected by the surgery, I would have to re-learn the basics. It would test the knowledge of the therapists, as well as the patience of Job!

First, I would have to learn to walk again. Days of total bed rest and the loss of balance made my first attempts at walking look like a giraffe's first ice skating lesson. My mind was barking the commands, "Go ahead, put those feet on the floor and move out!" But my legs were talking back: "I don't think so. Not in this lifetime!"

John Ruskin said, "If you want knowledge, you must toil for it; if good, you must toil for it; and if pleasure, you must toil for it. Toil is the law." Every inch of recovery was going to take God's grace and my grit. I knew it from the start. But I determined to let my stubborn roots grow deep into the "streams" and wait for the "fruit" that would be provided "in its season," as the psalmist promised.

But in between, I can assure you the leaf often "withered."

I took my first step like a toddler and then several others, one-by-one. My physical therapist was patient and very understanding. More than likely, he had heard about my spontaneous renditions of "How Great Thou Art," and didn't want to be in my vocal ensemble! Every morning at dawn, I would awaken the ward with my own medicated version of that great song.

And each day, I was wheeled into a room filled with curious stairways, railings, mirrors, and the coldest tile-covered floors this side of Anchorage, Alaska, in February! There, I became "as a little child" and trusted my therapist "shepherd" to "lead me in the paths of righteousness."

I was determined to regain the use of my stubborn limbs. It was more frustrating than painful, but I refused to give up. At times I felt as clumsy as a blindfolded elephant on the front row of a ballet, but every day brought tenacity to confused nerves and leg muscles. Soon, armed with a shiny new walker, I was stalking those antiseptic-smelling corridors, looking for someone to sing to.

In between my roving concerts, family members chauffeured me in a wheelchair.

I'll never forget one trip.

Dad was driving and I was praying! He suffered a slight distraction and in a nanosecond, I was driven into the wall—my head swathed in bandages, my eye covered with a pirate patch, trying to hold the ragged remnants of a hospital gown together. My only injury was a severely sprained pride. But I trusted him for another trip the next day.

Part of the recovery process is a refusal to submit to the situation.

I like the story of the Quaker who advertised that he would give 40 acres of rich farmland to anyone who was perfectly satisfied with what he had. A curious seeker approached him. The Quaker asked, "Are thee perfectly satisfied with what thee hast?"

"Yes," replied the seeker. With a sly wink and a wise word, the Quaker replied, "Then why doest thee want *this* land?"

Recovery includes a determination to move on. Though I was planted by the psalmist's "streams of water," I had to be determined to let the roots of my will grow toward it. I couldn't be satisfied to stay like I was—not in *this* land.

The Pain Before The Gain

Most often, the recovery process is painful. Sometimes that pain comes in the form of physical discomfort, and other times, it is emotional. Both are *real-to-the-bone*. But another aspect in recovery comes from planting our determination into the soil of the circumstance and waiting patiently for the results.

Being fed like a baby was another interesting interlude in my hospital stay. As I progressed, guiding hospital macaroni from the plastic tray to my crooked mouth was only slightly disastrous. However, the area around my bed did look like a junior high school cafeteria after a full-fledged food fight. But I was determined to win. Soon, with the help of understanding nurses and family members, I learned to feed myself. And I've been doing it very well, everyday since.

I once read that the great tenor, Luciano Pavarotti, was unsure whether he should be a teacher or a professional singer when he graduated from college. His father is said to have advised, "If you try to sit between two chairs, you will fall between them. For life, you must choose one chair." Seven years of determined study and stacks of frustration later, Pavarotti reached the Metropolitan Opera. Winners are willing to make the decisions no one else is willing to make.

You may be struggling with a recovery. Where to start? Start with a determination to win. Let your roots grow deep toward the ever-flowing streams of God's inexhaustible grace and the fruit will be born in "its season."

Going Home

Armed with a stubborn heart, tearing at my plastic ID bracelet, and laden with more plastic washbowls than I would use in a lifetime, I finally was loaded into a wheelchair for the trip to the lobby.

"Are you ready to go home?" Carol asked, while her face lit up like a beacon light at the grand opening of a furniture store. Our eyes met in a moment of wonderful joy, while our hearts sang silent hallelujahs. The Great Physician had, once again, created a miracle out of a mess!

At the hospital entrance, looking for all its worth like a Lincoln stretch limo, was our '66 Volkswagen Beetle. I entered it like a president—even to the point of giving the wheelchair nurse one of those parade waves.

The smell of spring filled my nostrils, my lungs, and my heart. It was Easter week and as we journeyed toward home, it seemed as if the Creator had personally planted flowers on every corner.

Adjusting Your Sights

Those sightings took a slight bit of adjustment, however. My left eye has been light sensitive since the surgery. But once I got used to the spring brightness, I reveled in the beautiful, warm day that God had planned.

I've often thought about that adjustment. There are times in our lives when our Heavenly Father uses a traumatic interlude to adjust our sight. Often, we live our lives slightly out of focus.

We set our sights on the most.

We look at the wrong.

We get our eyes on the worst.

We zero-in on the things of time instead of searching the horizons of eternity.

In providential love, our Heavenly Father, like an optometrist placing those oversized, metal goggles against our eyes, makes the adjustments and asks, "Which is clearer?" "This?" Or "This?" And each adjustment helps us see things clearer than we have ever seen them before.

I had been to the edge of eternity. I had walked closer to the grave than I had ever imagined. And the Giver of Sight had used a tender adjustment to make me see the things that mattered most.

New Heart, New Look

Since I had lost a tear duct in the operation, my left eye had to be partially sewn shut to keep the cornea from drying out. I wore a temporary patch but, with one good eye, I saw sights on that trip that I hadn't taken the time to see before. Those streets were well-known to me. I had traveled them during busy days of pastoral visitation. But something was different.

"Carol, was that flower bed always on the corner?"

"That grass is a beautiful shade of green!"

"The grocery store looks different. Did they remodel it?"

I was looking at my surroundings with new eyes and a new heart.

We pulled into the broken-cemented driveway of that fifty-year-old parsonage, and it was as if we were pulling into the White House. The Lord made sure that every available ray of sunlight was pointed at the house—the one that I often wondered whether I'd see again. It was His gracious way of saying, "I told you I'd take care of you."

The little white VW that we had "adopted" during the first year of marriage pulled to a stop beside a cabin cruiser in the yard. That boat was one of those bargain basement deals (with probably as much leakage as a real basement) that I had dreamed of. I only got to take one ride in it before my illness.

I thought I had to have it—as with many other gizmos in my life. Now, it was parked prominently and permanently in my backyard.

I stood beside it while my wife recorded the homecoming on one of those Kodak 126 Instamatic cameras that had all of the technological sophistication of a lead pencil.

Soon, that boat of my dreams would have a "For Sale" sign on it, and would become the financial nightmare in someone else's dreamworld. It didn't matter anymore.

I was determined not to live with the same old values.

Through surgery, therapy and partial recovery, I had discovered that life and living was of far greater significance than any material possession.

Written on a tombstone epitaph in an England cemetery were the words, "She died for want of things." Alongside, there was another tombstone: "He died trying to give them to her."

When you're learning to walk again, a first step is worth more than a Ferrari sports car.

When you're learning to feed yourself, a first bite is worth more than a Five-Star restaurant meal.

When you're determined not to succumb to your situation, nothing else really matters.

The Apostle Paul set his spiritual sights on his relationship with Christ and said the words that have echoed through the halls of time into our hearts:

I press on toward the goal to win the prize for which God has called me heavenward in Christ Jesus (Philippians 3:14).

Then Came Sunday

Easter Sunday is my favorite Sunday of the year. But no other Easter Sunday meant more to me than this one.

One week after my hospital release, I was to ascend the antique, wooden stairway of that centennial church, to the platform. I thought about it, as I pointed my Remington razor toward my face, for its journey into the unknown.

Suddenly the butterflies in my stomach were playing Ping-Pong with the vitamin pill I took at breakfast.

It wasn't so much knowing *what* I would say; it was knowing *how I looked.*

While I was in the hospital, a fellow clergy with as much tact as a runaway eighteen-wheeler with its wheels on fire made the remark in his deep-voiced "holy" tone, "Well, Jerry, I guess with that paralysis in your face, you'll have to think about leaving the ministry."

Matter of fact, I hadn't thought about it.

It hadn't even crossed my mind—until that awkward moment —that I might not be able to continue my pastoral ministry.

After he left the room (Thank the Lord!), I thought about it for a long time into the night. Sometime before dawn, I made the decision not to think about it anymore. God had called me. And God knew about this surgery a million years before He launched the first star in the galaxy.

My calling wasn't going to be held captive to the pitying whims of the thoughtless. I was a child of the Heavenly King, not an orphan of some earthly court.

I belonged because I belonged to Him.

That didn't make my Sunday morning glimpse in the mirror any less frightening, however. My hair was now about the length of the first fuzz of a six-month-old peach. The eye patch made me look like some character in Peter Pan, and when I smiled, my face looked like it was standing on its side.

I was afraid my congregation might ask for a refund when the offering plate was passed! The miracle of my standing, walking, and preparing to preach didn't enter my mind at that moment. It was only that awful vanity that causes us to look for ourselves first in a group picture!

I decorated myself as best I could, and with a little encouragement from a loving wife, I marched like General MacArthur back to the shores of my little church. This problem wasn't going to keep me out of the pulpit.

I was determined to win.

Whatever I said that Sunday, was semi-worthless compared to the sights in the audience. Over there was the Elmer Moore family. How they had opened their hearts to a young preacher and his wife! Elmer was the vice-chairman of the church board when I accepted the church's call. He had been a friend when, in their minds, some of the other members had backed a U-haul trailer up to the parsonage steps.

There was Ron Borgman. God had allowed me to encourage him in his own ministerial calling. But he always ended up ministering to me with a "wide-load" smile and a hug that would wring sawdust out of a California redwood.

The saintly and salty former missionary, Ione Driscoll, sat there with uncharacteristic tears chasing each other down her cheeks. I remembered the time when this dear, retired missionary to Sierra Leone had knelt alongside me in the late hours of an all-night prayer meeting, when everyone else had gone home.

She was at the altar near Dr. Chuck Pierson, then a young resident and later a medical missionary in West Africa, on that night when some of the dear church members held a prayer meeting prior to my surgery.

Nothing spectacular happened in that first service. And I was fortunate enough to make it up the platform stairs without falling on my face.

But the warmth of those people wrapped itself around my heart. The nods of their heads at the pitiful little sermon I delivered that day added to my determination to be all that I knew how to be for the cause of Christ and the advancement of His kingdom.

You'll never *get over* this situation in your life until you determine to get over it. I know that sounds a little bit like Yogi Berra's famous advice, "It's not over 'til it's over" but it's absolutely true.

The New Testament writer to the Hebrews said,

> *God is not unjust; he will not forget your work and the love you have shown him as you have helped his people and continue to help them. We want each of you to show this same diligence to the very end, in order to make your hope sure. We do not want you to become lazy, but to imitate those who through faith and patience inherit what has been promised* (Hebrews 6:10-12).

Get over it. Get going. And trust a God who will not fail. That's pretty good advice!

And that's the spirit that will take you from where you are to where you want to be. Be determined not to let your situation put your life in the loss column.

I had to have that kind of resolve as I began my ministry during those days of recovery.

Then I tried to play the piano.

FOUR

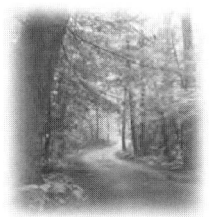

USE YOUR TRAUMA TO TEACH OTHERS

Praise be to the God and Father of our Lord Jesus Christ, the Father of compassion and the God of all comfort, who comforts us in all our troubles, so that we can comfort those in any trouble with the comfort we ourselves have received from God
(2 Corinthians 1:3-4).

Following the surgery, I had a solid gold song in my heart, but it just couldn't make its way to my fingers.

I'll never forget that day, in a little church in English, Indiana, when Dad said, "Why don't you start playing the piano for the congregational singing?" That had never occurred to me, nor had it occurred to me that God had given me any special musical gifts.

I remember that first song in the empty church. And I also remember the surprise in realizing that my 11-year-old fingers seemed to go where my mind and heart told them.

God had given me a natural "ear" to play the piano. After several days of practice, I played my first song. And I have been playing to the glory of God ever since.

Now, as part of the recovery process, I would have to learn how to play the piano all over again.

My first sermon after surgery came off without any noticeable incident. I wasn't thrown off the platform and no one tossed a pew Bible at me.

But I wasn't prepared for what happened when I tried to play the piano for the first time.

As I sat down to the piano, my right hand played on command but my left hand went "On strike!" It was as if one section of the orchestra suddenly picked up their instruments, stood up, and walked off the stage. The surgery had affected my motor skills and my brain wasn't sending the musical message to my left hand.

I soon felt like a child banging on piano keys, waiting for a voice of authority to tell me to stop. For me it was more frustrating than not being able to use a knife and fork.

Would I ever be able to play the piano again? First my smile, now my song. What was left?

The Gift That Keeps On Giving

A cousin by marriage, Lloyd Ganton, called me unexpectedly and told me there was a delivery truck on the way. It arrived. And so did a brand new spinet piano. The Lord used him to remind me (once again) that He wasn't through with me yet.

I first heard that suggestion while I was hovering in my spirit over the hospital bed during a full cardiac arrest. Now He seemed to re-inforce that message directly—and undeniably—to my heart.

The piano was a sign. And the Holy Spirit used it to put a new song in my heart.

Every day I would deliver a dose of musical discords to the best audience I ever had: my family. I truly believe that the same Great Physician who unstopped the deaf ears in Galilee, worked an opposite miracle on their ears! The sounds coming from that shiny new spinet piano were enough to make snakes squeal!

I also had a manual typewriter that Messrs. *Smith and Corona* had probably assembled personally during their first week of business. Along with the piano playing, I would sit at that antique typewriter for hours, pecking away at the keys, trying to get my fingers working again.

A few weeks later, my left hand began to come around. It was at least semi-obedient. The new song began to flow from my heart, into my fingers, and out through the sounding board of that piano. And the gift of that piano has kept on giving.

After all this time, my hands still don't pick up every musical signal my brain sends to them, but every song is dedicated to the Creator of Music. And He knows that no matter what I'm playing at the time, my heart is singing, "To God be the glory, great things He hath done."

Another musician summed it up:

> *I waited patiently for the LORD; he turned to me and heard my cry. He lifted me out of the slimy pit, out of the mud and mire; he set my feet on a rock and gave me a firm place to stand. He put a new song in my mouth, a hymn of praise to our God. Many will see and fear and put their trust in the LORD* (Psalm 40:1-3).

God Turns Our "Why's" Into "Wherefore's"

Christ is truly the High Priest who is touched by our infirmities. As we've noticed, on the Cross He asked the great question, "Why?" It was a word that kept echoing in my spiritual ears during those days. I asked it without spiritual doubt, but I asked it unreservedly and very humanly, as one new "learning experience" after another came my way.

But He has a wonderful way of turning our "Why" into a "Wherefore." Thirty days of recovery became a classroom where I would learn lessons that I would be privileged to teach others. My own "Why?" would connect to the questions of other seekers and become a "Wherefore."

I love the story of the little boy who walked into a pet shop to pick out a new puppy. Spotting a tiny one quietly lying in the back corner of a cage filled with frolicking pups, he said to the owner, "I want that one."

The owner tried to discourage him. "Son, you won't want that puppy. It was born with a defective hip. It won't be able to run and play with you like the others."

The little boy lifted his pant leg and pointed to a steel brace on his leg. "Maybe not, Mister, but I figure he'll need someone who will understand him."

I'll never forget the first time I walked into a parishioner's hospital room some months later. As a pastor, I was there to bring comfort and encouragement to someone who had been told about their terminal illness.

As I gripped his hand and began the conversation, the words fell from my mouth, "I know how you feel." In a moment, it all flashed back and I really did know how he felt.

I immediately added, "Believe me, Friend, I know how you feel. I've been there."

I really did. My Heavenly Father had taken a young pastor through a challenging orientation period to train him in understanding the hurts of others.

Now I knew what I was supposed to do with the victories over my own setbacks; I was to re-cycle them. My personal challenges were to be object lessons to teach the grace of the Almighty to those hindered by their own circumstances.

I was appointed to teach the lessons of healing over trauma.

Elmer Moore, the board member whose family had been so kind to us, was to become another of my students. A brain tumor was discovered early, but the surgery left him with partial facial paralysis. It was very uncomfortable to walk into his room and be greeted with a smile that nearly mirrored my own. But who would understand his feelings any better than I?

I breathed a prayer, mustered courage from the very human recesses of my heart, and opened the door. There he lay, having survived a life-threatening surgery and the removal of a virulent tumor, he was faced with a long physical and emotional recovery. Even as I asked about his condition, I knew how he felt deep inside. I understood the emotional battles that he would face. I knew how he would feel as he looked into the morning mirror. I knew the frustrations he would endure as he tried to eat a meal in a restaurant.

New Place, Same Face

Two years later, we accepted a pastoral call to Jackson, Michigan. And once again, the Lord had a student for me. A member of the congregation had suffered a severe stroke. And not surprisingly, one of the effects of the stroke was facial paralysis.

Divine appointment had once again brought a pastor who could understand, into the room of a patient who was struggling with understanding.

He even used that pastorate as healing ground.

Carol and I went to Jackson as pastoral candidates, with a new hope in our heart and a soft-pink bundle from heaven in our arms. Our daughter, Mandi, had been born perfectly whole in the August after my surgery, even though her mother had been given strong medication to stop labor in her back during my April surgery. Mandi's tiny presence was a giant incentive for me to complete my recovery.

We were given the assignment to candidate at Jackson Wesleyan Tabernacle. Because of the name, I visualized a large, stone-faced temple, filled with stuffy saints sitting on purple padded pews.

It wasn't like that.

We pulled into the dirt driveway alongside a church building that was smaller than a janitor's closet at the Crystal Cathedral. Since the doors were opened, I knew that the air conditioner was an item on the church board's agenda that had been "tabled" indefinitely.

The noise from the semis trucking down the by-pass next to the church all but drowned out my sermon. Maybe that's how I got the job!

It was a stuffy Michigan night, but that assignment would be a breath of fresh air to us.

The church had been started as a pioneer project. We spent the next decade as their pastors and marveled at their vision. Filling that tiny structure, we moved to two larger buildings, and what is now Trinity Wesleyan Church worships in a million-dollar building. I had the privilege of speaking to over 700 people on the first Sunday in the new facility. It was hard to hold back the tears, as I thought of how far the church had come from that night when we first met those dear folks.

During my ministry in Jackson, I started a fifteen-minute radio program called "New World." Months later, Carol and my sister, Ethel, who was now teaching in a Jackson school, joined me in launching a thirty-minute TV program called "First Day." A dear friend, Randy Sly, not only assisted us with the production but also served as co-host.

The TV program, with its Christian talk show format of news, music, and message, was a thrilling challenge. Every week I would have to raise $200 toward my "pay-as-you-go" agreement with the general manager. God gave me wonderful friends who shared the burden. Friends like John Stange, a young cereal manufacturing worker who traveled one hour from his home to assist us with taping the broadcast each Monday, and gave from his own funds to help support the broadcast.

Dick, the station floor manager, was anything but happy to have this "religious" program as his assignment. His occasional curses and routine frustrations slowly turned to curiosity and a personal search for faith. Carol and I shared Christ with him in a gentle but persistent way every week, and the barriers soon began dismantling. I'll never forget the look on his face when Dick Lee came to our parsonage door several months later. Once inside, with a smile that would have lit a Sahara desert night, he announced that he had given his heart to Jesus.

Later, his wife, Patti, would become my secretary and they both would bless our lives by their spiritual growth and willing service. Today, Dick Lee is blessing thousands of other lives as a station manager of a Christian radio station in a major metropolitan area.

There were others like Dick and Patti. And God sent all of them to us to assure our hearts that we had bona fide "teaching credentials" to help others in their hour of crisis.

Your Catastrophe Is A Classroom

A wise man, known for his contented living, was asked how he could be so happy. He replied, "It consists of making the right use of my eyes. I, first of all, **look up** to heaven and remember that my principle business *here* is to get *there*. Then I **look down** and call to mind how small a place I shall occupy on the earth when I die and am buried. I then **look around** and observe multitudes who are more unhappy than myself."

The Apostle Paul gave similar advice in his New Testament letter to Christians in Corinth (2 Corinthians 1:3, 4):

- **Look up:** *Praise be to the God and Father of our Lord Jesus Christ, the Father of compassion and the God of all comfort,*

- **Look down:** *who comforts us in all our troubles,*

- **Look around:** *so that we can comfort those in any trouble with the comfort we ourselves have received from God.*

There are several medicine bottles in our medicine cabinet that contain prescription medication unused from some previous illness. Please don't report us to the medical authorities, but sometimes we mark the illness on the bottles and use the medication when similar physical symptoms arise. I don't recommend that practice. And it's probably very unwise.

But in the same sense, we all have spiritual medicine bottles filled with leftover heavenly prescriptions that have sustained us in times of catastrophe. Those are the prescription remnants that we cannot only use at a later time, but remedies that can bring healing in the lives of others.

"I Get It!"

Catastrophe is a classroom where we learn the grace of a God whose hand doesn't shake in the winds of our times. It's a place where His Holy Spirit applies the spiritual balm of healing to our open wounds, and heaven's attendants are on duty 24/7 to hear our call.

It's also a place where we learn teaching skills that will, sooner or later, be used in helping others face their own catastrophes.

Sometimes the class time seems never-ending and the homework far too grueling.

But the "I get it!" look in the eyes of someone who has learned by our scars is worth every minute. Worth far more is the knowledge that we have a Heavenly Father who honors our persistence in spite of the problem and says, "Well done, Child. I know how much you hurt, but I want you to know how much I helped."

And someday, *we will fully know*.

On And On

Without making light of the horrible effects of substance abuse and the tremendous assistance given by support groups like Al-Anon, I still get a chuckle from someone's idea of a support group for long-winded preachers: "On-and-On."

God has let Carol and me use our trauma "on-and-on" to teach others how to cope with their catastrophe.

Often, as I would share my testimony with my parishioners, I could sense a comradeship that would blossom in courage to help those dear hearts face life at its worst. And I silently thanked the Lord for His providential leadership in my life.

I once got a card from a minister friend who was dying. In the card was a scripture quote from the anointed pen of a New Testament sufferer, the Apostle Paul. It started a thousand hallelujahs in my heart,

> *Now I want you to know, brothers, that what has happened to me has really served to advance the gospel. As a result, it has become clear throughout the whole palace guard and to everyone else that I am in chains for Christ. Because of my chains, most of the brothers in the Lord have been encouraged to speak the word of God more courageously and fearlessly* (Philippians 1:12-14).

And yet I couldn't help but notice the words, "most of the brothers in the Lord have been encouraged . . ." Some folk wouldn't be encouraged if an angel choir was sitting at their side humming *The Messiah* in their ear! But to those who will receive God's word of comfort, it's magnitude will far outweigh the calamity.

FIVE

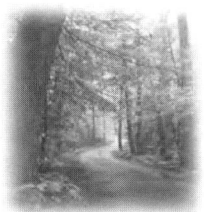

FOCUS ON THE DELIVERANCE

What, then, shall we say in response to this? If God is for us, who can be against us?
(Romans 8:31)

*I*t is a stirring picture. A seasoned sailor is in a tiny fishing boat on a storm tossed sea. The sailor is looking up toward angry clouds. The artist skillfully painted a prominent North Star right in the middle of the dark clouds. Underneath is the caption, "If I lose sight of that, I'm lost."

I received hundreds of cards and notes during my hospital stay. The greater percentage of them had a verse penciled below the signature: *We know that in all things God works for the good of those who love him, who have been called according to his purpose* (Romans 8:28).

If I had lost sight of that, I would have been lost!

The eighth chapter of Romans is filled with profound truth.

Two great gospel "bookends" begin and close the great chapter. Verses 1-2: *There is now no condemnation for those who are in Christ Jesus, because through Christ Jesus the law of the Spirit of life set me free from the law of sin and death,* and verses 38-39: *For I am convinced that neither death nor life, neither angels nor demons, neither the present nor the future, nor any powers, neither height nor depth, nor anything else in all creation, will be able to separate us from the love of God that is in Christ Jesus our Lord.*

The first speaks of the assurance of our salvation and the latter speaks of the assurance of our protection.

I claim both.

Sandwiched between the Cross and our coronation is His keeping. Ten thousand foes may come against our body, soul, or spirit—but He will not be shaken. John Bowrey wrote the 18th century lyrics we sing with gladness:

> *In the cross of Christ I glory, Tow'ring o'er the wrecks of time;*
> *All the light of sacred story, gathers round its head sublime.*
>
> *When the woes of life o'er take me, hopes deceive and fears annoy;*
> *Never shall the cross forsake me: Lo! it glows with peace and joy.*

What, then, shall we say in response to this? Paul asks. And then, like a heavenly TelePrompTer, the words scroll on the screen of our heart for us to recite: *If God is for us, who can be against us?*

Romans Eight also became a quiet sanctuary as I faced the next test.

Our family doctor, Jerome Mancewicz, who initially directed me to the right neurosurgeon advised me that the droop in my face, resulting from the surgery, could possibly be minimized. He referred me to the prestigious Henry Ford Hospital in Dearborn, Michigan. It was no accident that the doctor who was assigned my case was the chief neurosurgeon. God always had the A-team standing by!

Six months after my surgery, I was sitting with my wife in the office of Dr. Richard Knighton. He was retiring after an illustrious career in neurosurgery, and I was to be one of his last cases. (I never cease to be amazed at God's timing.) He greeted us warmly and explained surgical options for dealing with the results of the severing of my facial nerve, to remove the tumor.

He spoke gently and softly while he explained his proposal to do a surgical procedure. He planned to graft the nerve from the left side of my tongue to the facial nerve effected by the Acoustic Neuroma surgery. I missed some of the details while I thought about facing another surgery, but I heard one prognosis very clearly.

He spoke to both of us, but at this point his eyes focused on me. "I must say that I have performed this surgery on several people who depend on public speaking for their livelihood and, in each case, their speech was noticeably affected."

By then I had a FAMILY-size lump in my throat!

Trust God's Plan

In spite of the prognosis, there was a unified peace in Carol's heart and in mine. We talked about it as we made the trip back to our busy parsonage. The Lord Jesus Christ, our Senior Physician, hadn't failed us for a moment. He wouldn't usher me from the brink of disaster only to feed me to Satan's sharks now! The date was set and we rested in what we felt was God's plan.

An elderly member of one church where I pastored had a favorite scripture promise. It was such a favorite that she was known by it. Every sharing time, you could be sure that she would be quoting that beloved promise:

> *Trust in the LORD with all your heart and lean not on your own understanding; in all your ways acknowledge him, and he will make your paths straight* (Proverbs 3:5, 6).

Later in her life, her mind was dulled by senility. I would visit her, and on every visit I would have to explain who I was and what church I represented. She couldn't remember her friends' names anymore. But she never forgot the promise. Every time "church" entered the conversation, up came the promise: *In all your ways acknowledge him, and he will make your paths straight.* I can't tell you what an impression that made on my heart. God's promises are not dimmed by physical or mental damages. He can pierce the most troubled mind with a clear revelation of His care.

Carol and I had the privilege of laying the entire matter before His throne in prayer. We also had the privilege of making our plans for the return trip to Dearborn, with a quiet confidence that He would direct our paths.

The Same Old Gown

It was rather unnerving to be in a hospital bed, waiting for morning surgery again, but there I was—IN ONE OF

THOSE SAME OLD GOWNS, WITH A HAIRNET ON MY HEAD! After awhile the anesthesiologist came by for a chat and explained that in a few hours, I would be going to "Lullaby Land."

After he left, I reached for my Bible and realized that I had forgotten it.

Thank God for the Gideons! They have always been a favorite organization and the favoritism probably began that night. I reached into the bedside cabinet and pulled out a Gideon Bible that some faithful soldier had placed. I don't remember now what I read, but I do know it was promise enough for me to lay my head on a pillow, commit my life to the hands of my loving Heavenly Father, and sleep like a just-fed baby.

Believe The Best

Once again, the God-skilled hands of the surgeon did their work, and in a few hours I was back in my room.

I had been warned that the surgery's effect would not be immediate, so I looked into the mirror with little expectation. There was great expectation in my heart, however. I was trusting in God's plan—and His plans are trustworthy.

Since it was a teaching hospital, I soon became a glorified object lesson. Dr. Knighton and his merry band of "junior doctors" made a daily trek to my room. There, they would politely nod, write something or other in their spiral-wired notebooks, and place the details of my life in their crowded white pockets. I felt like sending them a bill for *my* services!

When I went back for a check up several weeks after my release, Dr. Knighton said, "Do you mind if I call some of my students in here?" Of course I didn't mind. Some of them had become my buddies by now.

"Say something, Jerry," he commanded.

I answered, "What would you like me to say."

Suprisingly, Dr. Knighton replied, "That's enough." Turning to his medical students, he said, "Ladies and gentlemen, I have performed this surgery hundreds of times in my career and these are the most successful results I have ever seen!"

Why wasn't I surprised? If God could give me a song in the storm, He could give me a way through the wilderness. *See, I am doing a new thing! Now it springs up; do you not perceive it? I am making a way in the desert and streams in the wasteland* (Isaiah 43:19).

Are you going through the wilderness—or do you still have "jet lag" from your last trip? Let me give you a word of advice: Focus on the deliverance.

I know it's human to focus on the *disaster*—to throw a pity party and gather worldly tools for coping with the adversity. But I'm inviting you to focus on the *deliverance*—to throw a celebration party in your heart, and acknowledge that God has this adversity under His infinite control.

God has already dug a stream in your desert!

Now . . .

- Claim His promise over the problem.
- Share a witness to His deliverance over the dilemma.
- Let your countenance display His victory.
- Start working toward bringing solutions to someone else's situation.

SIX

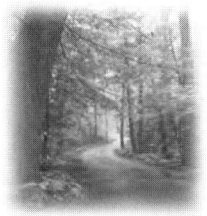

LEARN TO LIVE AGAIN

*Be strong in the grace that
is in Christ Jesus*
(2 Timothy 2:1).

"The winner says it may be difficult, but it's possible. The loser says it may be possible, but it's too difficult." I don't know where I got that advice, but it's good stuff. Everyone comes to the bottom of the mountain and momentarily looks up.

Some will then sit down in despair. Others will tie the shoelaces on their climbing shoes and begin the journey.

I chose to climb.

In his best-selling book, *God Has Never Failed Me, But He's Sure Scared Me to Death a Few Times* (Tulsa: Honor Books, 1995, p. 23), Stan Toler quotes the story of the great evangelist D. L. Moody crossing the Atlantic on a ship. The ship caught fire and a bucket brigade was formed to pass water from the ocean. One of the passengers on the brigade is said to have remarked to Moody, "Mr. Moody, don't you think we should retire from the line and go below to pray?"

D. L. Moody replied, "You can go pray if you want to, but I'm going to pray while I pass the buckets."

There's a time for faith and then there's a time for "faithfulness."

I chose to put faithfulness to my faith by returning to the work to which God called me. The nerve repair successfully minimized the droop of my mouth. And though I have weakness on the left side of my body, I have been speaking in public, singing, and playing the piano ever since. The climb hasn't always been easy, but the grace of Christ in my life has strengthened every step.

One doctor advised me that I would suffer bouts of depression for many years. *I have.*

A second doctor also advised me that my affected left eye would gradually degenerate. *It has.*

A third doctor said I might have to consider another line of work. *I haven't!*

What I have done is to learn to live again. And in the learning, I have discovered that a new life is possible for nearly everyone who has faced a trauma. My plan was quite simple.

1. Refuse to dwell on the difference.

A few weeks following my release from the hospital, Carol and I were on our way to California, for a *Campus Crusade for Christ* evangelism training session. I don't remember giving more than a passing thought to the fact that I would be facing hundreds of fellow participants in a strange new setting with my strange new face. With short hair barely covering surgical scars, my left eye sown partially shut, and with permanent numbness on the left side of my head, I guess I just thought they might need me for the cover of their next brochure!

It was a thrilling week in the beauty of the Arrowhead Springs training center. Somehow, I had convinced Carol to place our newborn in the hands of her grandparents and head west. Knowing her as I do, she probably went along to keep food off my chin. (Since the facial paralysis prevents me from feeling food particles on my face, she has given me cues with grace and charm.)

I even refused to dwell on the difference when I was appointed to team up with another pastor for door-to-door witnessing during that California training.

However, I did face one moment of awkwardness. Neither one of us was too crazy about this first attempt at "cold turkey" door-to-door witnessing stuff. Our awkwardness would soon turn to absurdity.

A pretty blond answered the door at the very first house. I had already made sure it was my partner's turn to speak at the first door. His opening words were, "Hello, Ma'am. My name is Jerry Brecheisen and this is . . . " His next words were, "No. That's not right. I mean, my name is . . . " And, to this day, that woman still doesn't know which one of us was the real Jerry Brecheisen!

But in the next hours, several people learned about Christ. And I learned that I still had a viable ministry.

2. Look for the humor in the horrible.

I also learned that humor was a great way to cope.

Even before my surgery, I was plagued with seeing the funny in just about everything. More than once I had bitten my lower lip to keep from smiling or laughing out loud when an "ecclesiastical absurdity" (dumb things in church) crossed my path. Now, since I only had feeling on the right side, it was possible to bite my lower lip and only feel half the pain!

Pastors don't have to look very far for the humorous.

I remember the time when a very haughty female funeral director took charge of a graveside service where I was officiating. And when I say, "took charge," I mean that.

I don't remember exactly when she lost control of the situation but it must have been pretty near the moment when she was "leading" the pallbearer-borne casket and her foot slid into the open grave. It was only my sanctification that prompted me to help her out!

Believe me, that battle to keep my composure ranks up there with the great struggles of history.

I have never been hesitant to refer to my differences, in a humorous way. But even in the humor, I refuse to dwell on them.

Part of a successful recovery is the process of moving on. It's a mind thing. It's a refusal to build nests for vultures of pity or resentment. It's not as though we don't have those thoughts. It's just a refusal to rent them space on the hard drive of our heart.

- God let it all happen.
- God loves us and accepts us as we are.
- God needs us in His greater work.

3. Consider what others are going through.

During the hours before my surgery, I had a chance to befriend another patient who was also facing surgery. He had a tumor directly on the brain. We were instant comrades because of the similarity. I don't remember his name but I remember that he, too, had a supportive and loving family.

We were unaware that we shared the same intensive care unit following our surgeries. Our families supported each other with kind comments and questions during our stay. My comrade's tumor was malignant, and the days following his release from intensive care were very difficult.

On the days I would return to the hospital for subsequent check ups, we would often meet. It was heartbreaking for Carol and me to hear his wife question why I seemed to be doing so much better than her husband. Whether it was the better part of wisdom, I don't know; but she had not been told that her husband's tumor was malignant.

As I would watch him struggle, I prayed for his strength, and silently thanked the Lord for sparing my own life. Ever since, I have had a keener eye for those facing adversity. It's not a pity glance. It's a gratitude glance. It's a heartfelt thanksgiving that my burden is far lighter.

Someone once told me about throwing "prayer darts" at people. It's both harmless and very rewarding. Often when I see another person struggling with a physical challenge, I will send a "prayer dart" in their direction—asking God to bring help to them and to their family. I know that He doesn't need to be reminded of their plight, but that mini-prayer time is a wonderful time of personal reflection on God's care for me.

4. Keep a God-perspective.

Keeping a proper perspective is important to coping with personal trauma. Of course, *our* personal tragedy seems to sail high above all others. But if we look closely and carefully at the conditions of others, we will discover that God has not brought an insurmountable problem into our own lives. The Apostle Paul reminded us of our common struggle,

> *No temptation has seized you except what is common to man. And God is faithful; he will not let you be tempted beyond what you can bear. But when you are tempted, he will also provide a way out so that you can stand up under it* (1 Corinthians 10:13).

The all-seeing, all-knowing, all-powerful, ever-present God of love has set a boundary around our infirmity. Time or testing will not take us a step farther than His sovereign purpose. He knows if our tolerance may be lower than that of another.

He can weave the helpless strands of our situations into a tight-fitting, strong tapestry that will withstand the traumas of life.

The same Lord who created ten *scillion* snowflakes, each with a unique pattern, knows us. The Creator of every inhabitant on planet earth, each with a totally unique set of fingerprints, knows his or her limitations. He will not allow a burden in our lives that He will not share.

5. Consider the alternatives.

I was surprised by the response of a parishioner whom I was visiting in the hospital. When I asked how she was, she responded, "I'm fine, Pastor, considering the alternative."

Each of us really is fine when we consider the alternatives.

A slight physical deformity is only a small burden to bear, considering the alternatives. If I hadn't survived the surgery, the emotional and financial loss for my family could have been severe.

I praise the Lord for the slight inconvenience. In fact, praise always helps to lift the load.

6. Don't let anyone steal your victory.

A guest speaker staying in our parsonage once asked my youngest daughter, Arianna, "Have you got the victory?" Her reply set me to thinking, as she said with a fallen countenance, "No Sir, I didn't take it." Here's a thought: How many times has someone else stolen our victory?

The colleague who came to my hospital room and became the first to remind me that I might have to change careers was a "victory thief." I've met others.

"What's wrong with your eye?"

If I had a dollar for every time that question was asked of me, I could almost pay a second's interest on the national debt. Since the tear duct was removed from my left eye during surgery, I have a "dry eye." If you've ever heard someone describe the impact of a drama or musical presentation with the comment, "There wasn't a dry eye in the house," you'll know I wasn't in the audience!

Several times a day, every day, I have to put artificial tears in that eye. Wind, tiredness, medications, or long hours of writing make it red and irritated. Overnight airplane flights are sometimes called a "red-eye." Every airplane flight I take is a "red-eye!"

I had to make a personal decision along the way that no one, or no-thing, would steal my victory. I refuse to play mind games with insensitive people who ask thoughtless questions about my physical appearance.

My simple response to the "eye question" is usually, "I had brain surgery." That usually settles the matter quickly, but sometimes I have to add, "I was a brain donor!"

I once saw a cartoon postcard that portrayed an elephant lying on its side, with a flock of large birds perched all over its obviously helpless body. The caption read: "Don't let the turkeys keep you down." The Old Testament prophet, Jeremiah, gave similar advice when he said to Israel, *Do not be afraid of them . . .* (Deuteronomy 20:1). Do you have a "Them?" Is there a person or a group that makes you feel uncomfortable with yourself? I thought about some "Thems" one day and jotted down a few words:

> I refuse to be afraid
>   Of Him, or She, or They.
> And I refuse to be alarmed
>   By what They All may say;
> For what are They, or Him, or She
>   But folks like You and Me,
> They certainly are nothing more
>   Than other folks like We;
> Yes, They are Us, and that's a fact,
>   With different bones and skin;
> And if you look back far enough,
>   They're prob'ly even kin.
> —JB

Refuse to be captive to comments or conditions—and go on!

7. Determine to get on with life.

A sign on the foyer of a church read,

> "Wake up, sing up, preach up, pray up and pay up, but never give up, let up, back up, or shut up, until the cause of Christ in this church and in the world is built up."

I could have remained hospitalized in my spirit, even after

my release from that Grand Rapids facility. But when I tore the plastic ID bracelet from my wrist, I bade farewell to the "patient." Since then, by the grace of God, He has allowed me to:

- Write over 100 gospel songs and choruses
- Host a weekly TV broadcast
- Host a daily radio program
- Release several vocal and instrumental albums of original songs
- Serve as managing editor of my denomination's magazine and producer of its international radio ministry
- Write, edit, or compile over thirty books
- Write hundreds of articles
- Speak to audiences nationally and internationally

Those aren't bragging points on a polished resumé they are memorial stones to the power and glory of God. If I had given in to my obvious differences and put my life on "PAUSE," I also would have missed the blessed friendships of some very special people around the world.

Whatever slight impact the Lord has allowed me to make on the lives of others is the result of a refusal to surrender to inner feelings of inferiority over some outward abnormality.

8. Refuse to abandon your goals.

I have personal goals that have been blossoming in my heart—even when the desert heat tried to dry my spirit.

Of course, some concessions have been necessary. I've decided (along with others) that I probably won't be chosen to model clothing in a Sears catalog.

And with some of the accompanying clumsiness that has dogged my motor skills, I probably won't be in the local ballet either.

But, I have been to Radio City Music Hall!

On the way to a tour in Israel, I spent several days in New York City, and was privileged to tour the NBC studios with a great friend, the late Don Brown. It's one of several sites the Lord has allowed me to see on my "revised journey."

A preaching assignment in Australia pounded another nail in the coffin of Satan's desire to wipe my sermon and song from the earth. The dear fellowship of my hosts, Lionel and Glenn Rose, and the gracious people of the "land down under," gave me further assurance that God had turned my life right side up!

There has never been a day in all the years of my ministry that the Devil hasn't tried to convince me to quit. His "You're-not-good-enoughs" and his "You-can't-do-thats" have been a dark cloud, following me throughout my journey. But one day, as I sat in a sidewalk cafe on the Gold Coast of Australia, on a reprise from several days of preaching, the Spirit of God reminded me of another verse to the song:

> *When through fiery trials thy pathway shall lie, My grace, all sufficient, shall be thy supply; The flame shall not hurt thee—I only design, Thy dross to consume and thy gold to refine.*

One Friday morning, a young man from Stanford University stood before an employer and asked for a part-time job. "The only opening I have now is for a typist," the office manager replied. The student immediately responded, "I'll take the job. But, if it's all right with you, Sir, I can't start until Tuesday."

On Tuesday, he reported for work. "Why couldn't you come back before today?" inquired his new employer. The young man answered, "Because I had to rent a typewriter and learn to use it!" The student was Herbert Hoover. His refusal to be a slave to his circumstance led him all the way to the White House.

SEVEN

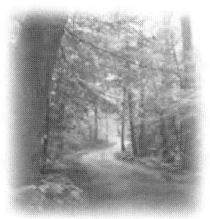

TURN YOUR WEAKNESS INTO STRENGTH

He sought God during the days of Zechariah, who instructed him in the fear of God. As long as he sought the LORD, God gave him success
(2 Chronicles. 26:5).

One philosopher wrote, "The block of granite which is an obstacle in the pathway of the weak, becomes a stepping-stone in the pathway of the strong."

During my pastorate in Jackson, Michigan, I was asked to be a fire department chaplain for the city fire department. The invitation seemed to be a "block of granite," but I quickly discovered that it was one of God's "stepping-stones."

Nearly one hundred firefighters and their families would soon become my second congregation. The chief was thrilled to have a volunteer who would be responsible for counseling the firefighters and their families, representing the department at funerals, ministering at the scene of major fires, and notifying next of kin in case of an injury or fatality. For three years, I would have the privilege of ministering in that capacity.

The first day was a childhood dream fulfilled. I was installed by the chief, given a gold chaplain's badge, and assigned "turn-out gear" (helmet, boots, and coat). The only drawback was the name on my white helmet and coat. Since the previous chaplain was a Catholic priest, I immediately became known as "Father DeMott."

Sitting in the cab of a ladder truck with its lights and sirens in motion was something I only imagined I would ever do. Along the way, I would discover that making bold steps would be rewarded by new and exciting opportunities.

About twice a month, I would stay all night at the fire station. It gave me an opportunity to get to know the firefighters and offered opportunities for on-site counseling. Through sharing my own struggles in response to their questions, they would learn of God's sustaining love and care.

My first night at the station was memorable. I wore a clergy shirt with a stiff, white plastic collar to distinguish me immediately at the scene of a fire (though I can't say I looked terribly distinguished in it). It was horribly uncomfortable – especially when I tried wearing it to bed.

At about 3:00 AM, the alarm sounded. After struggling with nervous insomnia throughout the night, I was barely asleep. But that alarm made me as alert as a purebred cat at a dog show!

Immediately, I jumped out of bed and into the night boots, with their canvas pants and suspenders attached. All I knew was that I was on the second level and I would have to get to the first floor in a hurry! So I made my clumsy way to the fire pole. Stations today are usually one story, so most firefighters will go their entire career without sliding a pole. I wish I could have!

Miraculously, I hit the pole and slid down to the gray cement floor. Then I remembered I had left my glasses upstairs. I soon learned that going back up the pole to retrieve them was not a good idea! Fifteen or twenty firefighters sliding down the pole were blocking my progress. I felt like it was raining people!

There were other challenges, as well. The chief had installed a siren and a magnetized rotating light in my personal car, so that I could respond to major fires from my home during the night. I'll never forget the night my parents were staying with us and the radio monitor in my room announced a fire. Trying to impress Dad, I quickly went to his room and asked if he would like to go with me to the fire. Soundly asleep, the word, "fire" was all he heard of that sentence. I think Dad's heart problems began that night.

We finally made it to the car—me in my clergy collar and Dad in his pajamas. I immediately put the revolving light through the window onto the roof. And several blocks later it somehow slid from the roof and stuck to my door on the driver's side. I remember feeling somewhat less pompous when Dad asked, "Jerry, are you sure that's where that light is supposed to go?"

Hundreds of stories would evolve from those three years. God let me touch the lives of hurting families, battered accident victims, and traumatized fire survivors. Days of busy pastoral ministry would be dotted with nights of fire and rescue runs. Each brought me a new awareness of my calling, and served as a reminder that God will use anyone in His service, as long as they are willing to let His strength override their weakness.

Give Yourself Wholly To God

Uzziah had to turn weakness into strength. During the prophet Zechariah's day, he was a "white-hat" righteous king in a succession of "black-hat" wicked kings over Judah. He was only sixteen years old when he replaced his godly father, Amaziah, but he became known for leading his people in a revival of love for Jehovah God.

At first glance, Uzziah had little going for him. His age certainly wouldn't garner much respect from the elders of his court. He had just started to shave, and the ink was still drying on his driver's license. But reading in this portion of God's Word gives us an idea of how he turned his weakness into strength.

First, he sought God. His success didn't come from his own power, but rather it came from his close proximity to the Divine.

> *He did what was right in the eyes of the LORD, just as his father Amaziah had done. He sought God during the days of Zechariah, who instructed him in the fear of God. As long as he sought the LORD, God gave him success* (2 Chronicles. 26:4, 5).

We begin to turn our weakness into strength when we give ourselves wholly to God. In the human, we don't even have enough inner resolve to walk by a "wet paint" sign without testing it!

Faith begins with the Father.

We will not conquer the kingdoms of doubt or adversity until we first seek God and do what is "right in the sight of the Lord." On the sleepy side of a Judean mountain, Jesus reiterated that truth in the greatest sermon ever preached. *Seek first his kingdom and his righteousness, and all these things will be given to you as well* (Matthew 6:33).

A decade later, I had to prove that promise. I was called to pastor a four hundred-member church in Roanoke, Virginia.

On my first day at the church I remember falling to my knees, alone and lonely behind the closed door of my office. Demons of doubt had camped in the room and began to sing their evil fireside songs about my inability.

They packed up and left when they heard the cry of my heart out loud. "I know this is way too big an assignment for someone who can't even offer a complete smile on his face. But, Lord, You called me here and this is where You will equip me for that call."

God faithfully used that surrender to His strength throughout a decade of ministry in the beautiful Roanoke valley. And previously, He had also given us another sweet bundle from heaven named Arianna. She and her sister, Mandi, sacrificially moved to a new school and new friends.

The victories were abundant. As our family gave ourselves wholly to God, He gave Himself to us in quiet communion. We were able to lead several other families to Christ. A childcare and early elementary school ministry were re-established (due largely to Carol's gifts and graces), with an enrollment of over 120 students (now over 150). The facilities underwent major renovations. And a host of Viginians became dearer to our hearts than human words could ever express.

Build On Your Natural Interests And Abilities

On one of those days filled with a hundred responsibilities and only about 10 tired ounces of strength left in my body, I jotted down some thoughts:

> I am only one.
> But I am one
> who has grasped the
> measureless promises of God,
> and touched the
> eternal currents of Pentecost.
> I am only one.
> But I am one
> who has embraced
> The One and Only,
> and found Him to be sufficient.
> —JB

While I have been privileged to use my interest in writing and editing as a ministry, file drawers contain the majority of my thoughts. In a music workshop taught by the esteemed songwriter, Bill Gaither, I heard him say that most of our writings will be between the Lord and us. It's so true! Much of my own writing has been "For His Eyes Only" and not for general circulation.

But that interest served as a personal therapy.

Uzziah turned his weakness into strength by building on his own interests and abilities. *Uzziah built towers in Jerusalem* (2 Chronicles 26:9). Each edifice was a monument of maturity. They not only occupied his time; they also served to give him credibility and personal confidence in his calling.

What can you do? Do what comes naturally. An honest search through your own gift inventory will reveal special abilities that can be used in overcoming trauma in your life, as well as bringing healing in the lives of others.

I like the story of the man who climbed a flagpole and began shouting at the top of his lungs. After being arrested for disturbing the peace, the judge asked him the reason for his actions.

"Your honor," he replied, "If I didn't do something crazy once in a while, I'd go nuts!"

Utilize The Strength Of Others

As mentioned before, Dr. Chuck Pierson was a parishioner who had been at that church prayer service the night before my surgery. A young surgical resident at the time, Chuck's life had been touched by a volunteer missions trip to Haiti. There, he watched the dedicated efforts of a Wesleyan missionary and sought out a Wesleyan church upon his return. I'm glad he found ours.

Chuck began a pattern of accelerated spiritual growth that soon was a blessing to the parsonage family and to the congregation of the church where we first pastored. After a long night in surgery, he could be found in one of the front pews on Sunday morning. His hunger for God's Word was evident. I shudder to think of the tiny portions of "soul food" he must have received from this rookie preacher. But he digested what he could, grew in his faith, and went on to bless thousands as a medical missionary in Sierra Leone, West Africa.

In the days and weeks following my surgery, Chuck could be found at the parsonage, doing the odd jobs that my partially-recovered strength would not allow. Often without notice, he would slip into the garage and pull out the lawnmower. We wouldn't even know he was there until we heard the lawnmower engine running. Another time, this busy surgeon came to the door and asked if he could paint the fence in our backyard. His acts of kindness, constant encouragement, and spiritual zeal blessed our lives.

But depending on others during my recovery was personally challenging. I had to understand that their strength supplanted my weakness.

Young King Uzziah turned his weakness into strength by his dependence on the skills of others. The Scriptures reveal this vital secret to his success: *In Jerusalem he made machines designed by skillful men for use on the towers and on the corner defenses to shoot arrows and hurl large stones. His fame spread far and wide, for he was greatly helped until he became powerful* (2 Chronicles 26:15).

Almost the entire chapter is marked with the mention of skillful artisans, agriculturists, architects, and armed warriors who helped his cause.

Utilizing the skills of others was always a struggle for me. From the very start, our young pastoral career had been nearly self-sustained. We hadn't learned the ministry of delegation, and my administrative skills were underdeveloped, to say the least.

One Saturday night prior to my surgery, after we had been to a week-long convention, we went to the church "office" (actually a small storage room off the platform) to print the bulletin. The manually operated Mimeograph had an ink well that was to be filled with messy black goo in anticipation of the Sunday bulletin. All of the mechanisms in that Mimeograph went into rigor mortis within a matter of minutes. And we spent the next agonizing hours trying to print bulletins. Each bulletin had to be hand fed, prayed over, and coaxed through the hellish machine. It was a pleasant evening!

Now during my recovery, I was dependent on others to print the bulletin and do most of my other jobs around that little church. I soon understood that all the while I had been doing "everything" in the church, I was robbing my parishioners of the development of their own gifts.

So many "recoverers" struggle with having to depend on the strength of others. Actually, there is no other way to turn weakness into strength, without utilizing the strength of the stronger.

Even the Strongest was ministered to. After Jesus' forty days of temptation in the wilderness, the Bible says, *Then the devil left him, and angels came and attended him* (Matthew 4:11).

Guard Your Heart

Uzziah's life didn't have a spiritual storybook ending. The prologue of the young king was a sad conclusion to a stellar preface.

> *But after Uzziah became powerful, his pride led to his downfall. He was unfaithful to the LORD his God, and entered the temple of the LORD to burn incense on the altar of incense* (2 Chronicles. 26:16).

He died a leper, physically and spiritually alone because he ceased to trust the Lord and arrogantly defied the ordinances of temple worship. The altar ceremony was reserved for temple priests, but Uzziah subverted them.

The days following a traumatic experience are equally crucial. Days and weeks of total dependence on the Lord and His family may be dangerously replaced with spiritual ease. The crisis is over. The victory has been temporarily accomplished. The recovery is in speed mode.

When others do your praying in crisis times, it may be easier to keep depending on them after the recovery process has matured. When every moment is in need of a scripture promise, it's far too easy to neglect the reading of God's Word after the initial cloud has lifted.

The recovered heart must be guarded against self-sufficiency. The legendary football coach, Vince Lombardi, once said, "Winning is not a sometime thing; it's an all-the-time thing. You don't win once in awhile, you don't do things right once in awhile, you do them right all the time. Winning is a habit. Unfortunately, so is losing."

EIGHT

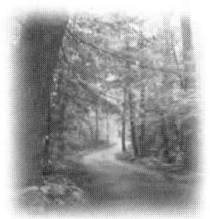

NEVER LOSE YOUR SENSE OF WORTH

*You made him a little lower than
the heavenly beings and crowned him
with glory and honor*
(Psalm 8:5).

A group of scientists was asked to estimate what it would take to duplicate a man's brain. They concluded that, if all the parts were transistorized and built to scale, it would take:

- A machine the size of the United Nations Building in New York
- A cooling system with an output equal to Niagara Falls
- A power source that would produce as much electricity as is used in homes and industry in the entire state of California

No wonder the psalmist was rapturous! When he thought about God's meticulous creation, his heart immediately sent rehearsal notices to the temple singers, sounded the ram's horn (an early prototype of the Sunday school bell), and gathered celebrants for a service of adoration and praise.

Why then, do debilitating illnesses often lower our self-esteem?

God Planned Your Life

Modern philosophers try to convince us that we are a terrestrial "OOPS!" and trip over God's revealed opinion:

> *My frame was not hidden from you when I was made in the secret place. When I was woven together in the depths of the earth, your eyes saw my unformed body. All the days ordained for me were written in your book before one of them came to be. How precious to me are your thoughts, O God! How vast is the sum of them!* (Psalm 139:15-17).

Think of it! Tiny, tadpole-like sperm battle the crashing currents of adversity in a furious freestyle swim toward a minuscule egg that God formed in His heart eons before He counted the brown particles of the Sahara sands. A miraculous union culminates in a unique cell that splits into equally unique parts.

And after approximately forty weeks of divine supervision and care, a tiny form pushes the "DOWN" button on a psychological and physiological elevator, through a birth canal so small that its tiny skull has to cave-in to make the journey, into the God-trained arms of an attendant. A child, formed with greater tenderness than the petal of a carnation, is born. And that solitary birth makes all of heaven sing "Happy Birthday," while several earthlings jostle each other to lay gifts at its feet.

You're a great miracle!

Partly cloudy skies often dim the view of our self-worth. But God isn't partly anything!

Infinite ages before the surgeons and technicians sat down over a cup of Grand Rapids-boiled coffee and discussed an operation on a fella named Jerry, God had seen the tender swipe of a cotton swab over the sight where the anesthesiologist would inject a careful sleep.

That surgery didn't come as a surprise. Heaven doesn't have to make the same adjustments we do. There is a master plan, drawn in love and signed in the blood of a Savior. Time or space does not limit our Heavenly Father. He was present at the first heartbeat and He'll be there at the last. In between, He has fashioned the days of our lives in infinite love and incomparable concern.

Sin carved ugly scars on the smooth surface of our days. Adam's rebellion paved the road to hospitals and funeral homes. God planned for us to live in a garden. Satan longed for us to make our residence in a garbage dump.

But with a cross of Calvary, the Lord Jesus Christ built a bridge over the dump. Though our Heavenly Father may allow us to go through times of trauma, He stands at the end of the tunnel with the keys to a kingdom where the word "pain" is never mentioned.

Sometimes God puts a heavenly umbrella over us to shield us from the storm. More often, He puts His arm around us *in the midst of the storm* and walks us through. Either way, He is glorified. Either way, His unfailing kindness caresses us and His inexhaustible power sustains us.

I like the story of the young man who took his girlfriend to the state fair. He got on one of those "guess-your-weight" scales that printed out a card which he read to his friend. "It says I am a dynamic leader, handsome, and much admired by women."

"Give me that card," the troubled girlfriend replied as she reached for the tiny piece of cardboard. "It probably got your weight wrong, too!"

God doesn't get anything wrong—especially His opinion of us!

You mean as much to Him after your trauma as you did before. He thought you were special then, and He hasn't changed His mind.

Trauma sometimes has a way of making us feel as significant as legs on a ladybug.

We are weaker than before.

We can't do some of the things we used to do.

Some who befriended us because of our abilities have abandoned us because of our inabilities.

But God looks past the pain and problem, into our soul. He sees someone worthy enough to merit the death of His only Son. He sees someone whose weakness is a good candidate for His strength. He sees a winner, even in a losing situation!

Hallelujah For The Holy Land

"Would you like to see my slides of the Holy Land?"

That question used to cause a footrace of cold chills up and down my spine. There is no right answer. If you don't wait for the slide show, you'll probably miss the dessert. If you stay, you'll probably miss a few hours of sleep. (I think it would help if the projectionist didn't insist on turning off the lights.) I often silently wondered why people would spend their savings on Dead Seas and barren wilderness.

Then I visited Israel.

The Dead Sea came to life and the barren Judean wilderness became a sight-sanctuary for my soul. There are already too many articles and books about Bible land journeys. I'll not add any more.

But I'll have to say that something happens to the human spirit when it walks where Jesus walked, sails where He sailed, kneels where He knelt, and laughs where He laughed.

The entire trip went too quickly for my tiny mind, and far too slowly for my tiny budget. But something happened to me at Calvary.

I stood with reverent awe at the place where, most Christians say, Jesus was crucified. I looked at the scarred hill and thanked the Savior for the stripes that brought my healing. I sang silent songs of praise to the Prince of Peace as I walked the cobble-stoned *Via Dolorosa*.

I have no desire to get into archaeological fistfights with anyone. I don't know the exact spot where the Son of God was born, died, or was buried. I only know that it must have been near the place where His Heavenly Father touched my heart afresh with His Spirit's anointing.

The Garden Tomb site did it for me.

There were many pilgrims near me, but in my heart I was alone there. At times, I listened to the scholarly Dutch evangelist with the world's greatest job: preaching the Resurrection to visitors at an empty tomb. The remaining time was spent wandering by myself around the quiet solitude of that garden.

Almost fearfully, I crossed the threshold of the empty tomb. There was something different about the place.

And then I knew why. It was the place of my hope!

I had walked the shoreline of death.

I had seen the light that evidently opens the doors to eternity.
I had faced life's great inevitability.

Now, here I was. At the very scene where the Spirit of a living God put a "VACANCY" sign over a borrowed tomb.

No sooner had the evangelist guide spoken the New Testament words, "I am the resurrection and the life," than the gospel goose bumps played tag under my skin.

I'm alive because He lives!

I could walk to the gates of death without fear, because a resurrected Lord is the Gatekeeper.

My sense of worth isn't based on the popularity votes of earthly panels; it's carved into the splintered remnants of an empty cross.

Paul said it: *By the grace of God, I am what I am.*

I may not be whole in body, but I am whole in spirit because of His indwelling Spirit.

My gifts may be limited by the debilitating effects of time, but the Eternal Giver of Life has taken residence in my heart, to take up the slack.

God Has The Last Word

The poet/philosopher, Henry Thoreau, penned a vivid description of humankind.

> *He makes histories of the universe, he directs the destiny of nations, but he does not know his own history, and he cannot direct his own destiny with dignity or wisdom for ten consecutive minutes.*

In my mind, I went back to that hospital room where "Job's comforter" advised me that my ministry was over.

At that moment, I would've had to borrow a ladder to put sunglasses on a centipede.

Called of God by the prayers of godly parents and grandparents. Yet finished. Washed up before I even started.

Says who?!

I like the e-mailed account of some medical records quotes that were actually dictated by physicians:

"By the time the patient was admitted, his rapid heart had stopped and he was feeling better."

"The patient is tearful and crying constantly. Also appears to be depressed."

"The patient is numb from his toes down."

"The patient refused an autopsy."

I can identify with the last one.

Doctors, lawyers, educators, and counselors don't have the final word. God does. *In the beginning was the Word, and the Word was with God, and the Word was God* (John 1:1).

After the medical attendants have thrown their bloodied gowns into the receptacles;

After the bailiff has turned out the lights in a ghostly courtroom;

After the counselor has rubbed an earth-wise chin and shaken a doubt-filled head;

After all is done and said, God will have the last word.

Long before the white-robed representatives of medical science had pronounced their woes on my future, my parents had placed my tiny form in the hands of a preacher grandfather and dedicated me to the will of the Kingdom.

Hell's bells would not chime over my demise until the final word was spoken by the One Who spoke the first.

Oh, and by the way—He hasn't spoken the final word in your life either!

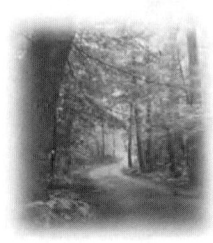

Contact Information

Jerry Brecheisen
P.O. Box 6073
Fishers, IN 46038
jerry@brecksong.com
www.brecksong.com

Other Books by Jerry Brecheisen

Looking at Life through My New Bifocals
When Life Doesn't Turn Out the Way You Expect
The Call to Contentment
Lead to Succeed
The Winning Dad
Psalms for Leaders
How to Prepare for your Baptism
26 Ways to Improve the Image of Your Church

Online Column

"Hope Above the Headlines"
www.brecksong.com

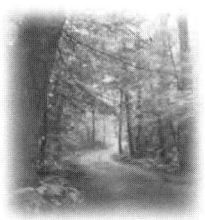

As Simple as A, B, C

God loves you very much. He longs for a relationship with you and has provided a way for you to know Him. The Bible outlines the steps to follow to enter a relationship with God. It's as simple as A-B-C.

Admit that you are a sinner. *For all have sinned and fall short of the glory of God* (Romans 3:23).

To sin is to disobey God on purpose. Sin may be revealed in words or actions, or it may be seen in an inner attitude of rebellion against God's will as revealed in His Word, the Bible. To admit that you are a sinner means to acknowledge your disobedience.

93

Believe that God sent Jesus to pay the punishment for your sin. *To all who received him, to those who believed in his name, he gave the right to become children of God* (John 1:12).

The penalty for your sin against God must be paid. But God loved you enough that He sent His own Son into the world to pay that penalty by sacrificing His life. Believing in God's loving plan for forgiveness is the next step to being reconciled to Him, becoming a part of His family.

Confess that you are sorry for sin and declare that Jesus Christ is now Number One in your life. *If you confess with your mouth, 'Jesus is Lord,' and believe in your heart that God raised him from the dead, you will be saved. For it is with your heart that you believe and are justified, and it is with your mouth that you confess and are saved* (Romans 10:9-10).

Accepting God's love and forgiveness means turning your back on your old way of living and turning your life over to Jesus Christ. It means agreeing with what God's Word says about Him. It also means following Him—putting Him first in your life—and seeking to grow in your relationship with Him.

Have you accepted Jesus Christ? Why not do it today? You can accept Him by praying a simple prayer like this:

> *Lord Jesus, I admit that I have sinned against You. I am sorry for my sin and I trust You to forgive me. I invite You to come into my life and help me to live for You all the days of my life. Amen.*

forgive us our sins and purify us from all unrighteousness (1 John 1:9).

Stand on God's promise, written in the Bible. He cannot lie. If God says that your past is forgiven—*it is!*

Step Three: Openly declare your new relationship with the Lord Jesus Christ.

Whoever acknowledges me before men, I will also acknowledge him before my Father in heaven (Matthew 10:32).

Tell someone about your decision. Ask your pastor about ways that you can openly acknowledge your faith.

Step Four: Grow by reading the Bible.

Like newborn babies, crave pure spiritual milk, so that by it you may grow . . . (1 Peter 2:2).

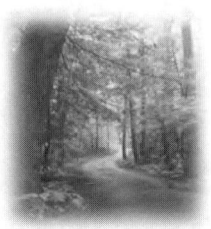

Steps To Your New Life

Step One: Know that you have invited the Lord Jesus Christ into your life.

I write these things to you who believe in the name of the Son of God so that you may know that you have eternal life (1 John 5:13).

Just as you are sure that you've had a physical birthday, you can be sure that you have had a spiritual birthday, that you have been "born again" by inviting Christ into your life.

Step Two: Trust God's promise of forgiveness.

If we confess our sins, he is faithful and just and will